Semantic-Pragmatic
LANGUAGE DISORDER

Charlotte Firth

Editor's Note

For the sake of clarity alone, in this pack we have used 'he' to refer to the child.

Published by
Speechmark Publishing Ltd, Telford Road, Bicester, Oxon OX26 4LQ
United Kingdom
www.speechmark.net

© Charlotte Firth & Katherine Venkatesh, 1999
First published 1999
Reprinted 2001, 2002, 2003, 2005

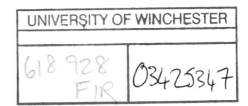
002-3342/Printed in the United Kingdom/1030
British Library Cataloguing in Publication Data
Firth, Charlotte,
   Introductory manual
   Part 1 Charlotte Firth, Katherine Venkatesh
   1. Speech disorders in children 2. Speech disorders in children – Diagnosis
   3. Speech therapy for children
   I. Title II. Venkatesh, Katherine
   616.9'2855'06

ISBN-10 for Part 1: 0 86388 326 5
ISBN-10 for complete set of 3 volumes: ISBN-10: 0 86388 329 X
ISBN-10 for Part 2: 0 86388 327 3
ISBN-10 for Part 3: 0 86388 328 1
Previously published by Winslow Press Ltd under ISBN 0 86388 240 4 (Part 1),
0 86388 241 2 (Part 2), 0 86388 242 0 (Part 3), 0 86388 203 X (complete set)

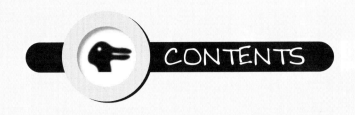

CONTENTS

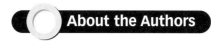

Charlotte Firth qualified as a speech & language therapist in 1989 from Leeds Metropolitan University. She has always worked in Yorkshire, initially with adults and children in clinic and hospital settings, but she began to specialize in paediatric work in 1990. In May 1990, she became a part-time research assistant at Leeds Metropolitan University, working with Dr Michael Perkins on a pilot study to investigate 'the use and comprehension of modal auxiliary verbs in children with a Semantic–Pragmatic language disorder'. In 1992, after another year working with children in schools and clinics, she took up her present post in Scarborough. She now works predominantly with special needs children in mainstream schools

Katherine Venkatesh (née Southwell) qualified as a speech & language therapist in 1986 from Leeds Metropolitan University. Since then, she has worked in North Derbyshire and Scarborough, specializing in working with children in a variety of settings. She has also qualified as a course tutor for the Derbyshire Language Scheme. Her involvement with this project arose from a chance remark in Summer 1996, when she offered to provide some pictures for her colleague Charlotte Firth's therapy programmes. At present, she is not working as a speech & language therapist as she is a full-time mother.

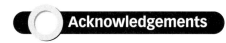 **Acknowledgements**

Firstly, we would like to acknowledge the help given by those who reviewed the first draft of the whole pack, Helen Harron, Mary Jones, Valerie Kingston and Mick Perkins.

Our thanks go also to our partners, Matt and Ashok, for all their support.

Charlotte would particularly like to thank John Lea for all his time, patience and technical expertise in producing the initial pack. She would also like to thank Mick Perkins for introducing her to the world of 'Semantic–Pragmatic' disorder.

In addition, Kathy would like to thank Rosemary Blakesley for the help and support she has always given.

Finally, thanks to the children and families who have provided us with the inspiration needed to produce this pack.

Charlotte Firth and **Kathy Venkatesh**

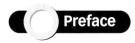 **Preface**

Semantic–Pragmatic Disorder: my first encounter with this term was as a student, just before my final exams. It was suggested that a question about the disorder would be likely to appear in our final year Speech Pathology examination. Following a hasty trawl through papers circulating at the time, I was relieved to find a question that summer (1989) which read: 'What might be the most relevant approach to intervention with a boy of ten with a Semantic–Pragmatic disorder?' I attempted to answer that particular question (I would enjoy reading my response now!) and my interest in the disorder was born.

Soon after qualifying, I worked as a research assistant at Leeds Metropolitan University on a project investigating how children with a Semantic–Pragmatic disorder understood and used modal auxiliary verbs. My knowledge and thoughts regarding the disorder started to develop and I began work that was later to form the basis for this resource pack. By summer 1996, I had developed the initial pack and Kathy joined me in the project. We redesigned the therapy ideas and adapted them to include Kathy's illustrations and handouts.

Today there is a great deal of published material regarding this language disorder. However, those in day-to-day contact with the children often seem frustrated by the lack of a simple framework to help identify, treat and manage this type of difficulty. I hope this resource pack will help meet this need to some degree. It does not purport to cover the wide range of theoretical models and therapy approaches that can be employed when working with individuals who have this type of disability. Most of the information in the pack has been acquired through time spent with these children and their families. The therapy ideas are merely a selection of the activities that have proved useful when working with children of this type.

Charlotte Firth
Malton, 1998

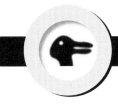

INTRODUCTION

A discussion regarding the disorder

Section 1

INTRODUCTION

here have been many papers, articles, reports and discussions in relation to Semantic–Pragmatic Disorder, and the subject still creates a great deal of interest. The following points summarize certain issues that recur concerning this disorder. Readers who anticipate some difficulty with the terminology used in this Introduction are advised to read first *Section 2 (Questions & Answers),* which will answer a number of the most frequently asked questions.

Interest in the UK in this 'new' disorder developed in the early 1980s. Several papers (including Culloden *et al*, 1986; Jones *et al*, 1986) were presented at the Invalid Children's Aid Nationwide Conference in 1986. These papers attempted to describe what did and did not constitute a disorder of this type. They also detailed how semantic, pragmatic (and syntactic) skills were affected in this type of language difficulty.

It soon became clear that it was not sufficient to detail characteristic features of this disorder, as the profile of the disorder changed over time. A characteristic pattern of semantic and pragmatic impairments became apparent. Initially, the child would be late to start speaking and would then use a great deal of echolalic language, often without comprehension. Later, the child would use relatively well formed language, the echoing would diminish but there would still be difficulties with comprehension. By around seven years of age, the child would understand more but have difficulties with social interaction (Shields *et al*, 1996). The child would speak inappropriately (Bishop & Adams, 1989), frequently change the topic and have difficulties maintaining a normal conversation (Adams & Bishop, 1989). When older, the child would have difficulties understanding the rules of social situations and conversations and interpret language very literally (Bishop & Adams, 1992, Kerbel *et al*, 1996). He would have continuing difficulties comprehending non-literal language, such as idioms: for example, "She flew across the room" (Kerbel & Grunwell, 1998).

Semantic–Pragmatic Disorder: Origins

Those who work with language-disordered children seek to classify linguistic problems, possibly in an attempt to plan therapy using informed judgements. Boucher (1998) feels that the use of Semantic–Pragmatic Disorder as a diagnostic category exists partly so that therapists can describe the child's difficulties and also to 'point the therapist towards goals and methods of intervention'.

Descriptive terms and labels change over time as ideas are refined and in the light of theoretical knowledge. There seemed to have been descriptions of what were semantic–pragmatic disorder-type difficulties without actually using this label. For instance, a paper entitled 'Language Without Communication: a Case Study', Blank *et al* (1979) described John (3 years 3 months). He did not interact with anyone other than his parents, but was age-appropriate in non-verbal areas.

1

He started to speak late, did not enjoy games such as 'peek-a-boo' and had sing-song prosody. His speech was clear and grammatically well formed.

Cromer (1981) felt that there was a need to identify difficulties in many areas, including cognition, phonology, syntax, *semantics* and *pragmatics*. This would then lead to a fuller understanding of language disorders. Rapin and Allen (1983) were also frustrated by the lack of means available to classify child language disabilities. They attempted to group these children into seven different syndrome types, one of which they named Semantic–Pragmatic Syndrome Without Autism. The development of this label was to start what has amounted to 15 years of discussion, debate and research into this type of language disorder. Rapin and Allen noted that these children produced syntactically well formed speech with good phonology, but had difficulty following conversations and had a striking inability to engage in communicative discourse.

Semantic–Pragmatic Disorder, Asperger Syndrome and Autism: How do they Differ?

This question has generated a great deal of research and (often heated) debate. Many argue that a child with Semantic–Pragmatic Disorder has a degree of autism and should not be identified as being apart or different from those with Asperger Syndrome or classic autism. Bishop (1989) attempted to describe autism, Asperger Syndrome and Semantic–Pragmatic Disorder as discrete disorders but with overlapping characteristics. A child with autism *is* likely to present with the typical characteristics of a Semantic–Pragmatic Disorder. Kanner (1943) recognized that disordered language was a cardinal symptom of infantile autism. He described autistic language as characterized by echolalia, metaphorical substitutions, transfers of meaning through analogy and generalization, literalness, pronoun reversals and verbal negations (Kanner, 1946). This is a familiar description.

Wing (1988) identified a triad of impairments in autism. She described a spectrum of deficits along three continuums of social functioning. The first of these was with social *recognition*, 'the ability to recognise that people are the most interesting and potentially rewarding features of the environment'. She felt that, at the milder end of the continuum, this was best described 'as a poverty of the grasp of the subtle rules of interaction and a lack of perceptiveness towards others'. Secondly, she described varying levels of difficulty with social *imagination and understanding*. This deficit inhibits the ability to understand the meaning and purpose of the actions of others, as it 'affects the ability to recognise what others may know or feel'. Thirdly, she detailed deficits in social *communication*, again at a milder level, this would impair 'the ability to recognise the needs of conversational partners'. Clearly, many children described as having a Semantic–Pragmatic disorder do exhibit these features to some degree.

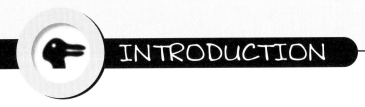

Perhaps a different diagnostic category evolved as children with milder difficulties did not fully satisfy the criteria for typical autism. Brook and Bowler (1992) felt, however, that focusing attention on the communication impairments and labelling them 'semantic–pragmatic' did not fully address these children's problems as any underlying degree of autism was then ignored. They felt that this may have happened when, for example, the child used eye contact or displayed prosocial behaviours. Autism was then disregarded whereas, if these features had been recognized as present but *inappropriate*, a more accurate diagnosis would have been made.

Boucher (1998) felt that, if we are to decide whether Semantic–Pragmatic Disorder is a valid diagnostic category, we should look closely at the way we describe both autism and specific language impairment. It may be possible then to decide whether it falls in, or perhaps between, the two categories. Boucher first described both autism and specific language impairment in terms of a 'syndrome' ('a unitary disorder [in which] diverse signs and symptoms stem from a single cause'). She stressed that semantic–pragmatic disorder could not form part of the autistic diagnostic category under this description as it would then be classified as 'mild autism'. This diagnosis would then be redundant as Asperger Syndrome is already used to describe mild autism. Nor could it be classified under specific language impairment if this is described as a syndrome, as we do not usually describe language disorders in this way since we know from our experience of acquired disorders that they do not have a unitary cause.

Boucher then went on to describe autism and SPD (Semantic–Pragmatic Disorder) within a 'spectrum of subtypes' concept. She noted that '… for SPD to be established as a distinct subtype of autism, clear and reliable differences as well as similarities would have to be established within the typical behavioural profiles of children with SPD as opposed to children with Asperger disorder kanner-type autism" (and other 'pervasive developmental disorders'). Semantic–Pragmatic Disorder could be a subtype of this type, and this is how Bishop (1989, mentioned above) tried to analyse the disorder.

Finally, Boucher described autism and Semantic–Pragmatic Disorder using the concept of a 'continuum of impairment'. She felt this idea was useful as it could then identify degrees of impairment in a range of developmental areas and individual profiles could be established. Equally, however, any specific diagnosis would be hard to establish using this model as there is scope for an almost endless range of variations. Autism and Semantic–Pragmatic Disorder would both then become nonentities (although we know that certain characteristics tend to group together). Boucher's final prediction was that Semantic–Pragmatic Disorder will prove to be a subtype of autism.

Perhaps if we look to the causes of what we will call 'autistic spectrum disorders' this may help with diagnosis.

Autistic Spectrum Disorders: Shared Deficits

If we consider what may cause the shared social and pragmatic impairments, this may reveal a common basis for these disorders. It appears that the majority of people with autistic spectrum disorders have some degree of difficulty processing sensory input, and what they see, hear, touch, smell and taste is not dealt with in the usual way. Information, for instance a sound, is received, but it is perceived in an unusual way. Boucher (1998) hypothesized that, 'SPD shares with both Asperger disorder and Kanner-type autism a specific deficit in information processing which impairs the registration and organization of complex experience, and to generate behaviour and to plan'.

We make sense of our world by analysing our experiences. We can deduce, infer and hypothesize by using, for instance, our judgement of the situations we are in, the people present and our knowledge of experiences we have already had. It is this ability, to draw information together at a 'central' level, that is impaired in autistic spectrum disorders. This skill usually starts to develop from birth and everyone differs in their level and type of 'central processing' ability. When there are significant deficits in this area, however, this can disrupt normal development. Frith (1989) stressed that, 'Just this particular fault in the mechanics of the mind can explain the essential features of Autism. The rest is secondary.'

Any characteristic feature of autism can be explained using this model. Examples might be the need for routine (necessary if it is difficult or even impossible to make sense of new information), restricted diets (again the threat of the unknown) or fear of new people (if it is hard to interpret their thoughts or how they might act).

How, then, does this difficulty in 'organising, drawing together information to make it coherent and meaningful' (Frith, 1989), affect someone's language skills?

Central Processing Skills and Linguistic Development

Semantic Skills

Semantics is the study of meaning in language (Crystal, 1985). A child develops his ability to attach meanings to words by gradually refining his concepts about his environment and the things he experiences. Early words are overgeneralized; for instance, initially 'male' may equal 'daddy' only, and then this term is applied for a short while to any man the child sees. As the child experiences more and develops concepts about the world, an increasingly complex vocabulary develops. If the child cannot draw information together to devise new ideas in this way, semantic development is unusual.

When a child has a central processing disorder there is a need for familiarity, resulting in a tendency for the child to develop first words that relate to his interests and personal needs. However, these words may not be very useful in a communicative sense. The child may, for instance, enjoy reciting words, for his own pleasure. There is less need to develop words such as 'mummy' if people are not a very important feature of the child's environment.

He may also remember words without having a true understanding of them. Jarrold *et al* (1997) studied a sample of 120 children with autistic spectrum disorders. They found that 'Children's scores on the WFT [a word finding test] were significantly higher than their scores on the BPVS [a test of receptive vocabulary].' Children with a Semantic–Pragmatic Disorder may learn many words in relation to particular areas, accumulated using their often excellent ability to memorize information. Paul (1987) mentions that 'Autistic children often develop large vocabularies and some take an obsessive interest in words and word meanings.' This is in contrast to normal development, when the child builds up a vocabulary through developing and refining his knowledge of the world around him, this type of development being through, and in response to, his everyday, communicative needs.

Later in the child's life this method of accumulating a vocabulary has an effect on the way words are interpreted. If a word is acquired by rote rather than through a developing understanding of the world around him, the child may find it hard to accept how words vary in their meaning, depending on the other words in the phrase or the situation they are used in. It will also be hard for the child to accept additional non-literal meanings of words and phrases.

Difficulties interpreting people's thoughts and situations, may mean that, for example, 'nice', said in a sarcastic tone, will be misconstrued. Metaphor and other similar uses of language may also confuse the child as he cannot consider the wider picture and use situational factors, including the person's tone of voice and experiential knowledge to interpret the words at a less literal level. The child may interpret certain words in one particular way. For instance, he may be annoyed if someone tries to say that 'bay' is the colour of a horse, when he has previously found that it relates to the seaside, or that 'on' can relate to the vertical plane (for instance, a clock can be 'on' a wall) when he has been taught 'on' in the horizontal sense. The child's inability to be flexible in this way will mean he may find it hard to accept these multiple word meanings.

Language skills are gradually built up following certain rules; for instance, words relate to one another and are classified in certain ways. Grammatical development also has a rule-based system by which it develops. If the child has not generated language using these systems, but has tended rather to memorize whole or part phrases, his speech will actually be delayed echolalia. It will then be hard for him to retrieve individual words as they may be 'hidden' within a learnt phrase. Word-finding difficulties can then occur.

Pragmatic Skills

Pragmatics is the study of the way language is used, the choices made and the constraints encountered when language is used for social interaction (Crystal, 1985). Individuals who have difficulties drawing information together to make

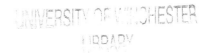

sense of the situations they are in are likely to have a pragmatic disorder. Other people will be confusing, and their actions potentially threatening, if it is difficult to construe what they may be thinking. This will be even more of a problem if the child finds it hard to process and understand speech. If he wants to converse, he will have little to guide him in his efforts. He may then use irrelevant language or dominate a conversation to feel more confident in his communicative attempts.

Non-verbal aspects of language, such as tone of voice and facial expression, will mean little to the child, as he will not have developed an understanding of these through experience. In short, this core inability to derive meaning by processing information at a central level can have anything from a mild to a devastating effect on pragmatic competence.

Syntactic Skills

Contrary to popular belief, it seems that children with a Semantic–Pragmatic Disorder do not always produce well formed, syntactically correct speech. As has been mentioned grammatical skills are normally built up and develop following a rule-based system. Children within the autistic spectrum tend to memorize language rather than develop it in this way. Where children described as having Semantic–Pragmatic Disorder seem to differ from those with autism and Asperger Syndrome is that there seems to be some correlation between the child's wish to be relevant and pertinent in conversation and the degree to which his speech becomes syntactically misformulated (although this seems to reach a peak at a certain age in these children). Consequently, those children with a lesser degree of the underlying deficit that causes the pragmatic disorder may produce phrases such as "The dog is barking to chase the cat" (a dog barking at a cat as he chases it) or "The maybe the if someone's inside the house and throw the key out outside, so might the man won't get in" (a man standing outside his house, who appears to have lost his keys).

This appears to be a result of the child struggling to produce a relevant response when he has only memorized whole phrases to help him do this. The child then tries to fit together segments or chunks of these phrases to formulate a good response (as he is partially aware of the needs of the listener and cares about their participation in the conversation to some degree). For instance, the following was produced as one continuous utterance: "They could be/a pool/ the boy's lying down/the girl's getting over/another pool" (a girl climbing out of a swimming pool oblivious to a boy in the pool who is shouting for help). The obliques in the quotation indicate where part phrases may have been used as the child attempted to get his message across.

In addition, the child may also exhibit 'false starts' as he tries to remember part and whole phrases; for instance: "After play, before play, I had it before, I had it before I had, I'll, I'll, see you after break."

Phonological Skills

Much has been made of the fact that children with a Semantic–Pragmatic Disorder do not have speech sound difficulties. If this is the case then it could be a result of the child memorizing speech he has heard, which, for the main part, is likely to be adult speech that is fully developed. Phonological skills usually follow a particular developmental route that is in step with all other areas of language development. Often children with Semantic–Pragmatic Disorder do not go through the usual developmental speech and language stages and this is given as a reason for the lack of normal phonological sound substitutions and/or disorders. However, processing difficulties can affect auditory skills and children may then internalize and copy speech as they have perceived it. The child may then produce rather unusual speech patterns, characterized by unusual, deviant phonological substitutions and structural abnormalities, such as producing only certain segments of words: for instance, "sman pa" (Postman Pat). Children may also produce very deviant phonological patterns and substitutions due to their processing disorder. These need to be appreciated as such and not necessarily as dyspraxic speech patterns (that is, expressive, motor programming difficulties).

Semantic–Pragmatic Disorder, Asperger Syndrome and Autism: Should We Use Separate Labels?

The above labels and several others, such as High LEvel Language Disorder (HLLD) (Hockey, 1989) appear to detail almost the same characteristics. Central processing difficulties produce a range of impairments, including linguistic impairment, but it is too simplistic to say that these form a range from mild to moderate. This cognitive disorder can affect a range of developmental areas, each in a variety of ways to differing degrees (the continuum concept). For instance, a child may have affected visual skills as a consequence of having a heightened perception of patterns or colours and then have a mild degree of this difficulty. This facet of the child's functioning in combination with his levels ability and disability in other developmental areas, form the clinical picture for that child.

Gagnon *et al* (1997) argue that there is little point in creating a new category of disability when there is already a "well-defined diagnostic category (ie. high functioning autism) whose symptoms coincide with those of semantic–pragmatic syndrome …". However, classic or 'Kanner type' autistic disorder is diagnosed when a child has a certain set of characteristics each of which he exhibits to a specific degree. Confusion arises when a child has the same characteristics, but some or all of thcsc typical features are exhibited to a milder degree. Such children then tend to have the most disordered areas of development labelled. Perhaps it is in response to this that a specific category (Semantic–Pragmatic Disorder) evolved, when evidently a certain subgroup of children had mostly linguistic deficits and less affected development in other areas.

We must not overlook, however, the fact that certain children can present with most of the features highlighted on a typical Semantic–Pragmatic checklist and not have the underlying cognitive deficits that also cause autism.

Cromer (1981) stresses: 'Some language-disordered individuals then, may be more profitably understood in terms of a deficit in the pragmatic component of their language system. This may be true of some autistic children as well as some children who do not share other features of autistic behaviour.' Rapin and Allen (1998) felt that some of the confusion in the differential diagnosis debate is a result of our tendency to classify at different levels of behaviour. The first and highest level is diagnostic, where 'autism' and 'specific language disorder' are both behavioural classifications. They stressed that language abilities form another, second level of classification and that, at this level, 'subtypes of the language deficits DLD [developmental language disorders] and autism/PDD [pervasive development disorder] overlap [and consequently] there is no justification for reifying SPD to the position of primary diagnosis'.

Certainly it appears that much of the confusion in 'labelling' arises from this point. It is quite nonsensical to debate whether two notions are the same or different if they describe separate levels of behaviour. We would be debating a similar point if we were trying to decide whether someone had tonsillitis or a sore throat. One is extremely likely to be a consequence of the other, but we must also be aware that it is possible at times to have a sore throat without it being due to tonsillitis.

A case in point would be a child with a specific word-finding difficulty. Such children often have severe pragmatic difficulties. For instance, they may say inappropriate things (as they cannot select words), join in conversations at the wrong time (as they start to speak when they have managed to think of what they need to say) and may deliver long monologues (as it may be easier to continue speaking once they have started). They may also develop rather repetitive interests and speech, as it will be easier to retrieve familiar words. They also clearly have semantic difficulties. This would demonstrate how a child could have the symptoms of a semantic and pragmatic disorder (the sore throat) without the underlying cause (the tonsillitis) being autism.

It is possible, however, that this group of children do not present with very early communicative problems, which the majority of children within the autistic spectrum exhibit. This does not mean, though, that it is incorrect to describe them as having semantic and pragmatic difficulties. Jarrold et al (1997) argue that autistic children's language deficits are cognitive rather than linguistic in origin. They note that, if they were linguistic, there would be phonological and articulatory difficulties present also, as these are 'almost always present in cases of specific language disorder'. However, as mentioned above, children with a central processing disorder can exhibit speech sound difficulties.

Firstly, these difficulties often present when the child has what appear to be specific difficulties processing the phonological components of speech. The child then makes imprecise copies of words and phrases he hears, becoming less precise the more he tries to memorize, so perhaps a single word may be relatively clear, but a rote learnt whole phrase or song will have many sound substitutions and 'muffled' pronunciations. Secondly, as the child often adopts a particular intonation pattern, for instance jerky syllable-timed speech, the sounds within the words may be articulated in an unusual way and speech will then sound odd at a phonetic level.

It seems therefore that it is almost impossible to differentiate children on the basis of the features of their particular developmental disorder. A possible solution could be to identify the *underlying cognitive deficit* and then use different labels to *describe* that child's particular difficulties. Then those that have mainly linguistic deficits would be labelled 'Semantic–Pragmatic', those with more significant social deficits but relatively intact language skills would be labelled 'Asperger Syndrome' and those with significantly affected skills in all areas of Wing's (1988) 'triad of impairments' could be said to have autism. Then a diagnosis of Semantic–Pragmatic Disorder would not exclude the underlying deficit, but merely serve to describe the child's linguistic functioning.

The other, much more generally favoured, solution (Aarons & Gittens, 1990) would be to call the underlying deficit 'autism' and describe individuals as having degrees and types of this. This may help the child and his family gain access to the support available to those with autism but, as Aarons and Gittens point out, 'the label "autism" has such negative connotations for some clinicians that they are reluctant even to consider it in relation to those children who are less seriously affected'. It is generally agreed, however, that one should not give a linguistic label to avoid having to give the possibly less acceptable diagnosis of autistic disorder.

◯ Identification of Children with Semantic–Pragmatic Disorder

Were these children identified at all 20 years ago? It is possible that their difficulties were misconstrued and thought to be a reflection of more general learning difficulties. Perhaps then they were educated in schools for children with moderate learning difficulties. The difficulties they experienced, especially if misinterpreted or mismanaged, may have led to behavioural difficulties. Rapin and Allen (1983) described a child with Semantic–Pragmatic Syndrome who had severe behavioural problems and was viewed as psychotic, his problems resembling childhood schizophrenia. Certain children may therefore have attended schools catering for behavioural problems.

Were these children referred to speech and language therapy? Perhaps not, but, as speech and language therapists have given more attention to pragmatic functioning, referrals have increased. Those referring clients to speech and language therapy are now more aware of communication impairments dealt with by therapists.

Nowadays we should attempt to identify children's semantic and pragmatic problems. We should also hope that, if these are the primary cause of their inability to access the curriculum, they are in the correct educational setting, which is one that understands and caters for their special educational needs.

◯ Summary

Children have semantic, pragmatic and other linguistic impairments for a variety of reasons. We need to take a holistic, multiprofessional approach when assessing a child with any type of developmental disorder to identify his specific difficulties. This will guarantee the correct educational and general support systems for the child and his family.

In certain cases there may be some justification in labelling the child's linguistic deficits only (for instance when a child has a word-finding difficulty affecting pragmatic skills). Otherwise, Semantic–Pragmatic Disorder should be accepted as a descriptive linguistic label that usually applies (to some degree) to any child with a central processing disorder.

Although displaying the range of difficulties associated with this disorder, certain children may have the most significant deficits in linguistic areas. However, if a 'diagnosis' of Semantic–Pragmatic Disorder is then given, we should recognize the common underlying cognitive disorder that most of these children share with those with autism or Asperger Syndrome. This is especially the case if we wish to plan appropriate intervention based on a true understanding of the child's difficulties.

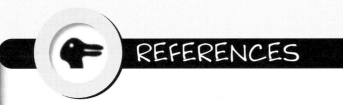

REFERENCES

Aarons M & Gittens T, 'What is the true essence of Autism?', *Speech Therapy in Practice* 5:8, 1990.

Adams C & Bishop DV 'Conversational characteristics of children with semantic–pragmatic disorder I: Exchange structure, turntaking, repairs and cohesion', *British Journal of Disorders of Communication* 24, pp211–239, 1989.

Amery H & Cartwright S, *First 100 Words*, Usbourne, 1987.

Amery H & Cartwright S, *First Thousand Words*, Usbourne, 1995.

Bishop DV & Adams C, 'Conversational characteristics of children with semantic-pragmatic disorder I: Exchange structure, turntaking, repairs and cohesion', *British Journal of Disorders of Communication* 24, pp211-239, 1989.

Bishop DV & Adams C, 'Comprehension problems in children with specific language impairment: literal and inferential meaning', *Journal of Speech and Hearing Research* 35, pp119–129, 1992.

Bishop DVM 'Autism, Asperger's syndrome and semantic–pragmatic disorder: Where are the boundaries?', *British Journal of Disorders of Communication* 24, pp107–121, 1989.

Blank M, Gessner M & Esposito A, 'Language without communication: A case study', *Journal of Child Language* 6, pp329–352, 1979.

Boucher J, 'SPD as a distinct diagnostic entity: logical considerations and directions for future research', *International Journal of Language and Communication Disorders* 33, pp71–81, 1998.

Brook SL & Bowler DM, 'Autism by Another Name? Semantic and Pragmatic Impairments in Children', *Journal of Autism and Developmental Disorders* 22, pp61–81, 1992.

Cromer RF, 'Developmental Language Disorders: Cognitive Processes, Semantics, Pragmatics, Phonology and Syntax', *Journal of Autism and Developmental Disorders* 11, pp57–73, 1981.

Crystal D, *A Dictionary of Linguistics and Phonetics*, Blackwell, Oxford, 1985.

Culloden M, Hyde-Wright S & Shipman A, 'Non-syntactic features of "semantic–pragmatic" disorders', *Advances in working with language disordered children*, ICAN, London, 1986.

Frith U, *Autism: Explaining the Enigma*, Blackwell, Oxford, 1989.

Gagnon L, Mottron L & Joanette Y, 'Questioning the validity of the semantic pragmatic syndrome diagnosis', *Autism* 1, pp37–55, 1997.

Hockey V, 'How to diagnose the child with "HLLD"', *Speech Therapy in Practice* 5:7, 1989.

Jarrold C, Boucher J & Russell J, 'Language profiles in children with autism: theoretical and methodological implications', *Autism* 1, pp57–76, 1997.

Jones S, Smedley M & Jennings M, 'Case study: A child with a high level language disorder characterised by syntactic, semantic and pragmatic difficulties', *Papers in Advances in Working with Language Disordered Children*, 17–21, ICAN, London, 1986.

Kanner L, 'Autistic disturbances of affective contact', *The Nervous Child* 2, pp217–250, 1943.

Kanner L, 'Irrelevant and metaphorical language in early infantile autism', *American Journal of Psychiatry* 103, pp242–246, 1946.

Kerbel D & Grunwell P, 'A study of idiom comprehension in children with semantic–pragmatic difficulties. Part II: Between-groups results and discussion', *International Journal of Language and Communication Disorders* 33, pp23–44, 1998.

Kerbel D, Grunwell P & Grundy K, 'A play-based methodology for assessing idiom comprehension in children with semantic–pragmatic difficulties', *European Journal of Disorders of Communication* 31, pp65–75, 1996.

Paul R, 'Communication', Cohen D, Donnellan A & Paul R (eds), *Handbook of Autism and Pervasive Developmental Disorders*, Wiley, New York, 1987.

Rapin I & Allen D, 'Developmental language disorders: nosologic consideration', Kirk U (ed), *Neuropsychology of Language Reading and Spelling*, Academic Press, New York, 1983.

Rapin I & Allen D, 'The semantic–pragmatic deficit disorder: classification issues', *International Journal of Language and Communication Disorders* 33, pp82–87, 1998.

Shields J, Varley R, Broks P & Simpson A, 'Hemispheric Function in Developmental Language Disorders & High Level Autism', *Developmental Medicine and Child Neurology* 38, pp473–486, 1996.

Wing L 'The Continuum of autistic characteristics', Schopler E & Mealbous GB (eds), *Diagnosis and Assessment in Autism*, Plenum, New York, 1988.

Also available from Speechmark

Working with Pragmatics

Lucie Andersen-Wood & Benita Rae Smith

Contains practical pragmatic teaching activities to develop communication skills. Offers an opportunity to explore this subject with confidence and to plan intervention programmes for effective management. Photocopiable assessment forms are included.

Autism: A social skills approach for children & adolescents

Maureen Aarons & Tessa Gittens

An excellent source of practical ideas on which to base programmes of intervention for children with autism. The content is primarily aimed at those working with children who have normal, or near normal, cognitive abilities, rather than those whose autism accompanies severe learning disabilities.

PETAL. Phonological Evaluation & Transcription of Audio-Visual Language

Anne Parker

PETAL is a tool for describing speech production patterns of children and adults in relationship to factors which may enhance or impede speech intelligibility. The approach used was originally developed for use with deaf children and adults, where the need to take account of audible and visible factors in speech assessment, development and conversation is a key factor. This boxed set includes photocopiable resources and 10 sets of illustrated cards.

Children's Phonology Sourcebook

Lesley Flynn & Gwen Lancaster

Lively and entertaining practical resource materials for speech and language therapists and others who work with young speech-disordered children can be found in this Winslow manual. Linking theory to practice, this is a user-friendly resource which encourages a thoughtful and creative approach to language remediation work.

Working with Children's Phonology

Gwen Lancaster & Lesley Pope

Successfully bridging the gap between theory and practice, this unique manual provides numerous creative ideas for lively and entertaining activities. It is a stimulating and essential resource which emphasises clinical approaches, contains clearly presented concepts, includes well illustrated original activities and examines advances in the analysis and description of phonological disorders.

Working with Children's Language

Jackie Cooke & Diana Williams

Well established and ever popular, this leading manual provides countless ideas along with a huge range of activities for language teaching. The combination of games, activities and ideas for developing specific language skills contribute to making this handbook a valuable resource for everyone working with children.

Early Communication Skills New Revised Edition

Charlotte Lynch & Julia Cooper

Containing a wealth of communication based activities, this practical resource will be invaluable to all professionals looking for fresh educational and therapeutic ideas in their work with preschool children and their parents.

Early Listening Skills

Diana Williams

This is a highly practical and user-friendly activity manual for professionals working with pre-school children who have underdeveloped listening skills associated with language delay, hearing loss or other communication difficulty.

Early Sensory Skills

Jackie Cooke

Creating a compendium of practical and enjoyable activities for vision, touch, taste and smell, this photocopiable manual is an invaluable resource for anyone working with children. The author outlines major principles and aims in six easy-to-use sections containing basic activities, everyday activities, games and topics to stimulate and develop the senses.

These are just a few of the many therapy resources available from Speechmark. A free catalogue will be sent on request. For further information please contact:

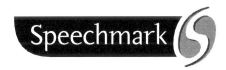

Telford Road • Bicester • Oxon OX26 4LQ • UK
Telephone: **(01869) 244644**
Facsimile: **(01869) 320040**
www.speechmark.net